ICU PEARLS

A Practical Guide for Critical Care Physicians

Dr Essam Abdelhakim

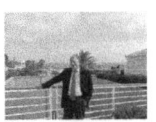

Copyright © 2024 Dr Essam Abdelhakim

All rights reserved

The characters and events portrayed in this book are fictitious. Any similarity to real persons, living or dead, is coincidental and not intended by the author.

No part of this book may be reproduced, or stored in a retrieval system, or transmitted in any form or by any means, electronic, mechanical, photocopying, recording, or otherwise, without express written permission of the publisher.

Cover design by: Art Painter
Library of Congress Control Number: 2018675309
Printed in the United States of America

CONTENTS

Title Page
Copyright
Disclosure
Introduction — 1
Chapter 1: Basics of ICU Management — 2
Chapter 2: Hemodynamic Monitoring and Support — 7
Chapter 3: Respiratory Support — 11
Chapter 4: Sepsis and Infections in the ICU — 17
Chapter 5: Neurological Emergencies — 21
Chapter 6: Renal and Electrolyte Disorders — 25
Chapter 7: Endocrine Emergencies — 30
Chapter 8: Trauma and Surgical ICU Management — 36
Chapter 9: Nutrition and Metabolism — 43
Chapter 10: Ethical and End-of-Life Issues — 49
CASE STUDIES IN ICU — 56
About The Author — 67

DISCLOSURE

Disclosure
This book has been created with the assistance of *Artificial Intelligence (AI) tools* and thoroughly reviewed and edited by the author to ensure clarity, relevance, and educational value.

While every effort has been made to provide accurate and up-to-date information, this content is intended solely for educational and informational purposes.

The author is a medical professional; however, the information provided in this book *is not a substitute for professional medical advice, diagnosis, or treatment.*

Readers are strongly advised to consult licensed healthcare providers or specialists for any medical concerns or conditions.

By using this book, **you acknowledge and agree** that the author shall not be held responsible or liable for any loss, damage, or harm whether physical, emotional, financial, or otherwise that may occur *as a result of the use or misuse of the information presented herein.*

INTRODUCTION

Overview Of This Book

This book, Critical Care Pearls: Essential Insights for ICU Physicians, has been meticulously crafted to provide you with practical, high-yield insights for managing critically ill patients. It is designed to be your go-to guide for tackling real-world ICU challenges efficiently and effectively.

The pearls in this book are derived from:

- Evidence-based guidelines.
- Expert consensus and years of clinical experience.
- Lessons learned from both successes and failures in the ICU.

Each chapter *covers key areas of critical care, such as respiratory support, hemodynamic management, sepsis, neurological emergencies, and ethical considerations. The pearls are concise, actionable, and focus on the most relevant clinical details.*

Whether you are a seasoned intensivist or a trainee just starting your ICU journey, this book aims to sharpen your clinical acumen and enhance patient care.

CHAPTER 1: BASICS OF ICU MANAGEMENT

1. Central Line Insertion

Clinical Scenario
A 55-year-old male presents with septic shock and requires central venous access for vasopressor administration. You prepare to insert a central line in the internal jugular vein.

Key Insight
Ultrasound guidance significantly reduces complications during central venous catheter placement compared to the landmark technique.

It enhances first-pass success and minimizes risks such as arterial puncture, pneumothorax, and hematoma.

Tips and Pitfalls
- **Preparation**: Ensure all equipment is sterile and readily available before starting. Perform a time-out to confirm the site and indication.
- **Ultrasound Use**: Always visualize the needle tip in real time to avoid accidental arterial puncture or posterior wall perforation.
- **Pitfall**: Avoid "blind" advancement of the wire; always confirm intraluminal positioning of the needle before proceeding.
- **Confirmation**: Verify catheter placement with post-procedure chest X-ray to rule out pneumothorax or

malpositioning.

Relevant Guidelines
- American Society of Anesthesiologists (ASA) and Society of Critical Care Medicine (SCCM) recommend the use of ultrasound guidance for central line placement to enhance safety and accuracy.

2. Arterial Line Placement

Clinical Scenario
A 70-year-old patient with acute respiratory distress syndrome (ARDS) requires continuous blood pressure monitoring. You decide to insert a radial arterial line.

Key Insight
The radial artery is the preferred site for arterial cannulation due to its superficial location and collateral circulation.
Ultrasound guidance improves success rates and reduces the risk of complications.

Tips and Pitfalls
- **Preparation**: Perform an Allen test or ultrasound assessment to confirm adequate collateral circulation in the hand.
- **Ultrasound Use**: Utilize short-axis visualization for initial needle insertion and long-axis for catheter advancement.
- **Pitfall**: Avoid excessive attempts in a single site, which increases the risk of hematoma and arterial spasm. Switch to another site if initial attempts fail.
- **Maintenance**: Secure the line firmly to prevent dislodgement, and monitor for complications like

ischemia or infection.

Relevant Guidelines
- The American College of Chest Physicians (CHEST) supports ultrasound guidance for arterial line placement to minimize complications and improve success.

3. Ventilator Management

Clinical Scenario
A 60-year-old female with pneumonia and hypoxemic respiratory failure is intubated and placed on mechanical ventilation. Initial settings include volume-controlled ventilation.

Key Insight
For most patients, lung-protective ventilation with a low tidal volume (4–6 mL/kg of predicted body weight) reduces ventilator-associated lung injury (VALI). Maintaining plateau pressures below 30 cm H_2O is crucial for lung protection.

Tips and Pitfalls
- **Initial Settings**: Start with FiO_2 at 100% and titrate down based on oxygenation (target SpO_2 88–92% in ARDS). Adjust PEEP to improve oxygenation while avoiding overdistension.
- **Pitfall**: Avoid over-reliance on FiO_2 for oxygenation; optimize PEEP and recruit alveoli instead.
- **Monitoring**: Regularly monitor arterial blood gases and ventilator waveforms to detect auto-PEEP, asynchrony, or overdistension.
- **Weaning**: Assess readiness for extubation daily with spontaneous breathing trials.

Relevant Guidelines
- The ARDS Network protocol recommends lung-protective ventilation strategies, emphasizing low tidal volumes and limiting plateau pressures.

4. Sedation And Analgesia Strategies

Clinical Scenario
A 45-year-old male with severe trauma is intubated and requires sedation and analgesia for mechanical ventilation and pain control.

Key Insight
The goal of sedation in critically ill patients is to maintain comfort, reduce agitation, and ensure synchronization with the ventilator while avoiding oversedation, which can prolong mechanical ventilation and ICU stays.

Tips and Pitfalls
- **Choice of Agents**: Use short-acting agents like propofol or dexmedetomidine for sedation. For analgesia, opioids like fentanyl are preferred due to rapid onset and short duration.
- **Sedation Protocols**: Implement daily sedation interruptions and use validated scales like the Richmond Agitation-Sedation Scale (RASS) to guide titration.
- **Pitfall**: Avoid benzodiazepines as first-line agents unless indicated (e.g., alcohol withdrawal) due to their association with delirium.
- **Monitoring**: Regularly reassess pain using tools like the Behavioral Pain Scale (BPS) or Critical-Care Pain Observation Tool (CPOT).

Relevant Guidelines
- The Society of Critical Care Medicine's (SCCM) Pain, Agitation, Delirium, Immobility, and Sleep (PADIS) guidelines emphasize multimodal approaches to sedation and analgesia, prioritizing non-benzodiazepine agents and daily sedation assessments.

CHAPTER 2: HEMODYNAMIC MONITORING AND SUPPORT

1. Interpreting Advanced Hemodynamic Parameters

Clinical Scenario
A 65-year-old male with sepsis remains hypotensive despite adequate fluid resuscitation. You initiate advanced hemodynamic monitoring using a pulmonary artery catheter.

Key Insight
Advanced hemodynamic monitoring provides insights into preload, afterload, and contractility.

Parameters such as central venous pressure (CVP), pulmonary artery wedge pressure (PAWP), cardiac output (CO), and systemic vascular resistance (SVR) guide therapy and help differentiate between types of shock.

Tips and Pitfalls

- **CVP**: Use as a trend rather than an absolute value to assess fluid responsiveness. A low CVP suggests hypovolemia, while an elevated CVP may indicate fluid overload or right-sided heart failure.
- **PAWP**: Elevated PAWP (>18 mmHg) typically indicates left-sided heart failure or fluid overload. Low PAWP suggests hypovolemia.
- **Cardiac Output**: Low CO with high SVR suggests cardiogenic shock, while low CO with low SVR points to

distributive shock.
- **Pitfall**: Avoid over-reliance on static parameters (e.g., CVP or PAWP alone) for guiding fluid resuscitation. Dynamic measures like pulse pressure variation or stroke volume variation are more reliable.

Relevant Guidelines
- The Surviving Sepsis Campaign recommends the use of advanced hemodynamic monitoring in complex cases to guide resuscitation efforts.

2. Managing Shock

Clinical Scenario
A 70-year-old female with a history of coronary artery disease presents with altered mental status, hypotension (BP 85/50 mmHg), and a lactate of 4 mmol/L. You need to differentiate between shock types to initiate appropriate therapy.

Key Insight
Shock is categorized into hypovolemic, cardiogenic, distributive, and obstructive, each requiring a specific approach to management.
Early identification and targeted treatment are crucial to improve outcomes.

Tips and Pitfalls
- **Hypovolemic Shock**: Prioritize fluid resuscitation with crystalloids (e.g., Ringer's lactate) and consider blood products if hemorrhage is the cause. Avoid excessive fluid administration to prevent dilutional coagulopathy.
- **Cardiogenic Shock**: Optimize perfusion with inotropes

- (e.g., dobutamine) and afterload reduction if indicated. Early consultation for mechanical support (e.g., intra-aortic balloon pump or ECMO) may be lifesaving.
- **Distributive Shock**: Treat the underlying cause (e.g., sepsis, anaphylaxis). Start norepinephrine as the first-line vasopressor in septic shock. Administer corticosteroids in refractory septic shock.
- **Obstructive Shock**: Relieve the obstruction (e.g., thrombolysis for massive PE, pericardiocentesis for tamponade). Avoid excessive fluids, which can worsen outcomes in cases like pulmonary embolism.
- **Pitfall**: Misdiagnosing the type of shock can lead to inappropriate therapy (e.g., giving excessive fluids in cardiogenic shock). Use hemodynamic monitoring and clinical assessment together.

Relevant Guidelines

- The American Heart Association and European Society of Cardiology recommend tailored management strategies for shock, emphasizing early identification and targeted interventions.

3. Pearls On Vasoactive Agents: When And How To Use

Clinical Scenario
A 55-year-old male in septic shock has a mean arterial pressure (MAP) of 55 mmHg despite adequate fluid resuscita
tion. You decide to start a vasopressor.

Key Insight
Vasoactive agents are vital in managing shock, with each agent targeting specific pathophysiological mechanisms.

Norepinephrine is the first-line agent for septic shock, while dobutamine is preferred for cardiogenic shock with low cardiac output.

Tips and Pitfalls

- **Norepinephrine**: Start at 0.01–0.03 mcg/kg/min and titrate to maintain MAP ≥65 mmHg. It provides potent vasoconstriction with minimal effect on heart rate.
- **Epinephrine**: Useful as an adjunct in septic shock refractory to norepinephrine or in anaphylactic shock. Monitor for tachycardia and hyperlactatemia.
- **Dobutamine**: Ideal for low cardiac output states. Avoid in severe hypotension without vasopressor support.
- **Vasopressin**: Consider in refractory septic shock as a second-line agent. Use at fixed doses (e.g., 0.03 units/min) to avoid adverse effects.
- **Pitfall**: Avoid high doses of vasopressors without addressing the underlying cause of shock, as this can lead to ischemia and organ damage. Always ensure adequate intravascular volume before initiating vasopressors.

Relevant Guidelines

- The Surviving Sepsis Campaign and the American College of Cardiology recommend norepinephrine as the first-line vasopressor for septic shock and highlight the role of vasopressin and epinephrine as adjuncts.

CHAPTER 3: RESPIRATORY SUPPORT

Case 1: Ards Management Pearls - Ventilator Strategies And Adjunctive Therapies

Clinical Scenario

A 42-year-old woman with no significant past medical history is admitted to the ICU with acute respiratory distress syndrome (ARDS) following a severe viral pneumonia. She is on a mechanical ventilator with settings adjusted for ARDS. Despite the ventilator support, her oxygenation remains suboptimal.

Key Insight

ARDS management requires lung-protective ventilation strategies aimed at reducing ventilator-induced lung injury.

The key strategies include low tidal volumes (6 mL/kg ideal body weight), plateau pressures <30 cm H2O, and maintaining adequate PEEP to prevent alveolar collapse.

Tips and Pitfalls

- **Tip**: Use prone positioning early in ARDS patients with moderate to severe hypoxemia (PaO2/FiO2 < 150), as it improves oxygenation and reduces mortality.
- **Pitfall**: Avoid high tidal volumes or excessive inspiratory pressures, as these can exacerbate ventilator-induced lung injury and worsen outcomes.

Relevant Guidelines

- The **ARDS Network** trial supports the use of low tidal volume ventilation (6 mL/kg) and optimal PEEP to improve survival and reduce ventilator-associated complications.
- **Surviving Sepsis Campaign** guidelines recommend the use of adjunctive therapies such as inhaled vasodilators (e.g., nitric oxide) and neuromuscular blockers in severe ARDS cases to improve oxygenation.

Case 2: Non-Invasive Ventilation - Indications And Troubleshooting

Clinical Scenario
A 68-year-old man with a history of chronic obstructive pulmonary disease (COPD) is admitted to the ICU for acute exacerbation. He is mildly hypoxic with increased work of breathing and moderate respiratory distress. The team is considering non-invasive positive pressure ventilation (NIPPV).

Key Insight
Non-invasive ventilation (NIPPV) is a first-line therapy for COPD exacerbations, acute cardiogenic pulmonary edema, and other conditions causing acute respiratory failure without the need for intubation.
Early use can avoid intubation and improve outcomes.

Tips and Pitfalls
- **Tip**: Ensure the patient has a secure airway and is cooperative before starting NIPPV. Monitor closely for improvement in respiratory parameters (e.g., blood gases, respiratory rate).
- **Pitfall**: Don't delay intubation if there is failure of NIPPV (persistent hypoxemia, hypercapnia, or respiratory distress despite adequate settings) or if the patient is not tolerating the mask.

Relevant Guidelines
- The **American College of Physicians (ACP)** recommends the use of NIPPV in acute respiratory failure due to COPD exacerbation or heart failure

to avoid the complications of invasive mechanical ventilation.
- The **ATS/ERS guidelines** emphasize careful patient selection for NIPPV, including assessing consciousness, ability to protect the airway, and the severity of respiratory distress.

Case 3: Weaning From Mechanical Ventilation - Strategies And Pitfalls

Clinical Scenario
A 75-year-old man has been on mechanical ventilation for 10 days following a large ischemic stroke with respiratory failure. His respiratory parameters are improving, and he is being considered for weaning. The ICU team is debating the optimal approach for extubation.

Key Insight
Weaning from mechanical ventilation is a gradual process that requires careful assessment of respiratory function, readiness to breathe spontaneously, and adequate cough strength.

The primary strategies include spontaneous breathing trials (SBT) and gradual reduction of ventilator support.

Tips and Pitfalls
- **Tip**: Perform a spontaneous breathing trial (SBT) using CPAP or pressure support to assess the patient's ability to tolerate breathing without the ventilator. If the patient maintains adequate oxygenation and ventilation for 30 minutes, they are typically ready for extubation.
- **Pitfall**: Avoid rushing the weaning process; the patient

may not be ready for extubation if they fail the SBT. Assess for factors such as adequate cough, adequate muscle strength, and stable hemodynamics before making a decision.

Relevant Guidelines

- The **American College of Chest Physicians (ACCP)** and **American Thoracic Society (ATS)** guidelines recommend using SBTs as part of the weaning process, with a trial duration of 30 to 120 minutes, and careful monitoring during this period to identify any signs of respiratory distress or failure.
- **Surviving Sepsis Campaign** also emphasizes assessing weaning readiness early in the ICU stay to optimize recovery and avoid unnecessary delays in extubation.

Summary Of Key Points For Chapter 3: Respiratory Support

1. **ARDS Management:**
    - Use lung-protective ventilation strategies (low tidal volumes, optimal PEEP, plateau pressures <30 cm H2O).
    - Prone positioning and adjunctive therapies like neuromuscular blockers may be beneficial in severe cases.
2. **Non-invasive Ventilation:**
    - Indicated for COPD exacerbations and cardiogenic pulmonary edema.
    - Ensure patient cooperation, monitor for failure, and consider intubation if necessary.
3. **Weaning from Mechanical Ventilation:**

- Spontaneous breathing trials (SBT) are essential for assessing readiness for extubation.
- Avoid early extubation in patients who fail the SBT or have underlying respiratory weakness.

CHAPTER 4: SEPSIS AND INFECTIONS IN THE ICU

1. Early Recognition And Management Of Sepsis And Septic Shock

Clinical Scenario
A 65-year-old female presents to the ICU with fever, hypotension (BP 85/50 mmHg), tachycardia (HR 110 bpm), and altered mental status. Laboratory tests reveal leukocytosis (WBC 18,000/µL), lactate of 4 mmol/L, and a positive urine culture.

Key Insight
Sepsis is a life-threatening organ dysfunction caused by a dysregulated host response to infection.
Rapid identification and treatment, including early fluid resuscitation and antibiotics, are critical to improving outcomes.

Tips and Pitfalls
- **Early Recognition**: Use the *qSOFA* (Quick Sequential Organ Failure Assessment) criteria—hypotension, altered mental status, and tachypnea—to identify high-risk patients.
- **Fluid Resuscitation**: Start with 30 mL/kg of crystalloid fluids within the first 3 hours for hypotension or lactate ≥4 mmol/L. Monitor for signs of fluid overload.
- **Antibiotics**: Administer broad-spectrum antibiotics within the first hour of sepsis diagnosis. De-escalate therapy once pathogen sensitivities are known.

- **Pitfall**: Delaying source control (e.g., abscess drainage, removing infected lines) can lead to treatment failure. Address the source promptly.
- **Hemodynamic Support**: Initiate norepinephrine if MAP is <65 mmHg after adequate fluids. Add vasopressin or epinephrine as needed.

Relevant Guidelines
- The Surviving Sepsis Campaign recommends early recognition and immediate treatment, including the "1-hour bundle," with emphasis on fluids, antibiotics, and hemodynamic monitoring.

2. Antimicrobial Stewardship In The Icu

Clinical Scenario
A 55-year-old male admitted for septic shock from pneumonia improves after 48 hours of broad-spectrum antibiotic therapy. Cultures reveal Streptococcus pneumoniae sensitive to ceftriaxone.

Key Insight
Antimicrobial stewardship aims to optimize therapy by selecting appropriate agents, dosing, and duration while minimizing the emergence of resistance and adverse effects.

Tips and Pitfalls
- **De-escalation**: Narrow therapy based on culture and sensitivity results to reduce unnecessary exposure to broad-spectrum antibiotics.
- **Duration of Therapy**: Follow evidence-based guidelines; most infections, such as community-acquired pneumonia, require 5–7 days of antibiotics.
- **Pitfall**: Overprescription or prolonged therapy

increases the risk of Clostridioides difficile infection and resistance.
- **Monitoring**: Regularly reassess the need for antibiotics, guided by biomarkers like procalcitonin and clinical response.

Relevant Guidelines
- The Infectious Diseases Society of America (IDSA) emphasizes prompt de-escalation and appropriate duration of therapy to balance efficacy and resistance prevention.

3. Managing Multidrug-Resistant Organisms (Mdros)

Clinical Scenario
A 72-year-old male in the ICU develops ventilator-associated pneumonia (VAP). Sputum cultures reveal Acinetobacter baumannii resistant to carbapenems.

Key Insight
Infections with MDROs are challenging and require precise antimicrobial therapy guided by susceptibility patterns. Preventing their spread within the ICU is crucial.

Tips and Pitfalls
- **Infection Control**: Implement strict contact precautions, including hand hygiene and isolation, to prevent cross-contamination.
- **Combination Therapy**: Use combination therapy (e.g., colistin with meropenem) for severe infections caused by carbapenem-resistant organisms.
- **Pitfall**: Avoid empiric use of last-resort antibiotics

(e.g., colistin, tigecycline) unless necessary, as this accelerates resistance.
- **Antimicrobial Cycling**: Rotate commonly used antibiotics to reduce the selective pressure for resistance.
- **Prevention**: Strategies such as minimizing ventilator days, maintaining central line bundles, and judicious use of antibiotics are essential.

Relevant Guidelines
- The Centers for Disease Control and Prevention (CDC) recommends a multi-modal approach, including antimicrobial stewardship and infection control measures, to combat MDROs in critical care settings.

CHAPTER 5: NEUROLOGICAL EMERGENCIES

1. Intracranial Pressure Management

Clinical Scenario
A 45-year-old male involved in a motor vehicle accident presents with a Glasgow Coma Scale (GCS) score of 7. CT scan reveals a large subdural hematoma with midline shift. The patient shows signs of increased intracranial pressure (ICP), including bradycardia, hypertension, and irregular respirations.

Key Insight
Elevated ICP is a life-threatening condition requiring rapid intervention to prevent herniation.
Management focuses on reducing ICP while maintaining cerebral perfusion pressure (CPP).

Tips and Pitfalls
- **Head Position**: Elevate the head of the bed to 30° to enhance venous outflow. Avoid neck hyperflexion or rotation.
- **Osmotic Therapy**: Use hyperosmolar agents such as mannitol (0.25–1 g/kg IV) or hypertonic saline to decrease ICP. Monitor serum osmolarity and electrolytes closely.
- **Sedation and Analgesia**: Ensure adequate sedation to reduce metabolic demand and prevent agitation.
- **Pitfall**: Avoid aggressive hyperventilation; while it

reduces ICP transiently, prolonged hypocapnia can cause cerebral ischemia. Maintain PaCO$_2$ at 30–35 mmHg only temporarily if herniation is imminent.
- **Neurosurgical Consultation**: Promptly consult neurosurgery for definitive management, such as decompressive craniectomy or hematoma evacuation.

Relevant Guidelines
- The Brain Trauma Foundation recommends targeting ICP ≤22 mmHg and maintaining CPP between 60–70 mmHg in traumatic brain injury patients.

2. Status Epilepticus: Rapid Intervention Strategies

Clinical Scenario
A 28-year-old female with a history of epilepsy presents with continuous generalized tonic-clonic seizures for the past 15 minutes. She has not responded to her usual antiepileptic medication.

Key Insight
Status epilepticus is a neurologic emergency with a high risk of morbidity and mortality.

Rapid intervention to terminate seizures and prevent neuronal injury is essential.

Tips and Pitfalls
- **First-Line Therapy**: Administer benzodiazepines (e.g., lorazepam 4 mg IV at 2 mg/min; may repeat in 10–15 minutes if seizures persist).
- **Second-Line Therapy**: If seizures continue, start antiepileptic drugs such as fosphenytoin (20 mg PE/kg IV), valproate, or levetiracetam.
- **Refractory Status Epilepticus**: Initiate continuous IV infusion of midazolam, propofol, or pentobarbital if

seizures persist despite second-line therapy.
- **Pitfall**: Delay in administering second-line agents increases the risk of refractory status epilepticus. Ensure timely escalation of therapy.
- **Supportive Care**: Secure airway, maintain oxygenation, and monitor for metabolic derangements (e.g., hypoglycemia, electrolyte imbalances).

Relevant Guidelines
- The Neurocritical Care Society and the American Epilepsy Society emphasize early use of benzodiazepines, followed by appropriate second-line agents.

3. Brain Death Assessment: Key Clinical And Legal Aspects

Clinical Scenario
A 60-year-old male with a massive intracerebral hemorrhage is unresponsive with fixed and dilated pupils. He has no corneal or gag reflexes, and apnea testing shows no spontaneous respiratory effort. The family inquires about brain death determination.

Key Insight
Brain death is a clinical diagnosis requiring careful assessment of neurologic function to confirm irreversible cessation of all brain activity.
It has profound clinical, legal, and ethical implications.

Tips and Pitfalls

- **Preconditions**: Ensure the absence of confounding factors such as hypothermia (<36°C), sedative drugs, or metabolic abnormalities.
- **Clinical Examination**: Confirm unresponsiveness, absence of brainstem reflexes (e.g., pupillary, corneal, oculocephalic), and lack of spontaneous breathing during an apnea test.
- **Ancillary Tests**: Consider additional tests (e.g., cerebral angiography, EEG) if the clinical exam is equivocal or cannot be completed.
- **Pitfall**: Premature declaration of brain death without ruling out reversible causes (e.g., drug intoxication) can lead to legal and ethical complications.
- **Family Communication**: Provide clear and compassionate explanations of the process and implications of brain death.

Relevant Guidelines

- The American Academy of Neurology (AAN) provides detailed protocols for the clinical determination of brain death, emphasizing a systematic and thorough approach.

CHAPTER 6: RENAL AND ELECTROLYTE DISORDERS

1. Acute Kidney Injury: Causes, Prevention, And Management

Clinical Scenario
A 72-year-old male with sepsis from a urinary tract infection (UTI) develops oliguria (urine output < 0.5 mL/kg/hr) and rising serum creatinine (Cr 2.5 mg/dL, baseline 1.0 mg/dL). His blood pressure is low despite adequate fluid resuscitation, and his lactate is elevated.

Key Insight
Acute kidney injury (AKI) is common in critically ill patients and is associated with increased mortality.

Early recognition, appropriate fluid management, and avoidance of nephrotoxic agents are key to prevention and management.

Tips and Pitfalls

- **Prevention**: Ensure adequate hydration, particularly in high-risk patients (e.g., elderly, those with sepsis or hypotension). Avoid nephrotoxic drugs such as NSAIDs and contrast agents, or minimize their use in high-risk patients.
- **Identification**: Use a rise in serum creatinine (≥0.3 mg/dL within 48 hours or ≥50% increase) or reduced urine output (oliguria or anuria) to diagnose AKI.
- **Management**: Focus on optimizing perfusion—address hypotension, correct fluid and electrolyte imbalances,

and manage underlying causes (e.g., infection, obstruction).
- **Pitfall**: Over-resuscitation with fluids in patients with AKI, particularly in those with pre-existing heart failure, may lead to pulmonary edema. Monitor closely for signs of fluid overload.
- **Monitoring**: Continuous monitoring of urine output, renal function (creatinine, BUN), and electrolytes is crucial for timely adjustments.

Relevant Guidelines
- The KDIGO (Kidney Disease: Improving Global Outcomes) guidelines recommend early identification and treatment of AKI, emphasizing avoiding nephrotoxins, ensuring adequate perfusion, and using nephrology consults when necessary.

2. Indications For Renal Replacement Therapy In The Icu

Clinical Scenario
A 68-year-old woman with severe AKI secondary to septic shock fails to respond to fluid resuscitation and vasopressors. Her serum potassium is 7.2 mEq/L, and her creatinine is 6.5 mg/dL. She is becoming increasingly acidotic, and urine output remains <10 mL/hour.

Key Insight
Renal replacement therapy (RRT), including hemodialysis or continuous renal replacement therapy (CRRT), is required when conservative

management fails to correct life-threatening complications of AKI, such as hyperkalemia, acidosis, and fluid overload.

Tips and Pitfalls
- **Indications for RRT**: The classic indications are the *AEIOU* mnemonic:
  - **A**cid-base abnormalities (severe acidosis)
  - **E**lectrolyte abnormalities (e.g., refractory hyperkalemia)
  - **I**ntoxication (e.g., lithium, ethylene glycol)
  - **O**verload (e.g., pulmonary edema despite diuretics)
  - **U**remia (e.g., encephalopathy, pericarditis)
- **Pitfall**: Delaying RRT can lead to irreversible organ damage. Initiate RRT early if any of the aforementioned indications are met.
- **Dialysis Modalities**: CRRT is preferred in unstable patients due to its continuous and gentler nature, while intermittent hemodialysis is more suitable for hemodynamically stable patients.
- **Vascular Access**: Ensure adequate access (e.g., central venous catheter) for RRT and consider temporary dialysis access if long-term access is not yet available.

Relevant Guidelines
- The KDIGO guidelines recommend timely initiation of RRT based on clinical judgment and laboratory parameters, particularly when patients develop life-threatening complications of AKI.

3. Managing Common Electrolyte Abnormalities (E.g., Hyperkalemia, Hyponatremia)

Clinical Scenario
A 58-year-old male with chronic kidney disease and diabetes develops severe hyperkalemia (serum potassium 7.5 mEq/L) following the initiation of an ACE inhibitor. He is lethargic and has peaked T-waves on his ECG.

Key Insight
Electrolyte abnormalities, particularly hyperkalemia and hyponatremia, are common in critically ill patients.

Prompt correction is vital to prevent life-threatening complications, such as arrhythmias and seizures.

A. Hyperkalemia

Tips and Pitfalls
- **Immediate Management:**
    - **Stabilize the myocardium**: Administer calcium gluconate 10% (10 mL IV over 2-3 minutes) to protect against arrhythmias.
    - **Shift potassium**: Use insulin (10 units IV) with glucose (25 g IV) to drive potassium into cells. Alternatively, nebulized albuterol (10-20 mg) can be used.
    - **Remove potassium**: Initiate dialysis if potassium is ≥6.5 mEq/L or if other treatments are ineffective.
- **Pitfall**: Do not rely on calcium alone to treat hyperkalemia—it only stabilizes the myocardial membrane and does not lower potassium levels.

Relevant Guidelines
- The American College of Cardiology (ACC) recommends rapid treatment of hyperkalemia in the

presence of ECG changes or potassium >6.5 mEq/L.

B. Hyponatremia

Tips and Pitfalls
- **Identification**: Hyponatremia is defined as serum sodium <135 mEq/L. Causes include volume depletion, SIADH, and heart failure. Symptoms range from mild (nausea, headache) to severe (seizures, coma).
- **Treatment Strategy**:
    - **Acute, symptomatic hyponatremia**: Raise sodium slowly with hypertonic saline (3% NaCl), targeting a correction rate of no more than 6–8 mEq/L in 24 hours.
    - **Chronic, asymptomatic hyponatremia**: Correct underlying causes and monitor sodium levels. Avoid rapid correction to prevent osmotic demyelination syndrome.
- **Pitfall**: Rapid correction of hyponatremia, particularly in chronic cases, can lead to neurologic complications, including central pontine myelinolysis.

Relevant Guidelines
- The American Society of Nephrology (ASN) and the European Society of Intensive Care Medicine (ESICM) emphasize the need for slow and controlled correction, particularly in cases of chronic hyponatremia.

CHAPTER 7: ENDOCRINE EMERGENCIES

1. Diabetic Ketoacidosis And Hyperosmolar Hyperglycemic State

Clinical Scenario
A 45-year-old female with poorly controlled type 1 diabetes presents with confusion, nausea, and abdominal pain. Her blood glucose is 650 mg/dL, arterial pH is 7.1, bicarbonate is 15 mEq/L, and her serum ketones are elevated. She is diagnosed with diabetic ketoacidosis (DKA).

Key Insight
Diabetic ketoacidosis (DKA) and hyperosmolar hyperglycemic state (HHS) are serious acute metabolic complications of diabetes that require rapid intervention.

While both conditions share hyperglycemia as a common feature, they differ in their pathophysiology, clinical presentation, and management.

Tips and Pitfalls
- **DKA Management:**
    - **Fluids**: Start with 1–2 liters of isotonic saline (0.9% NaCl) over the first hour to restore intravascular volume and improve perfusion.
    - **Insulin**: Administer an intravenous (IV) insulin infusion (0.1 units/kg/hr) once serum

potassium is >3.3 mEq/L. Avoid a bolus of insulin, as this can lead to rapid changes in serum potassium.
- **Electrolyte Management**: Monitor potassium levels closely. Even if potassium is initially normal or elevated, it can drop dramatically once insulin is administered, requiring potassium replacement.
- **Bicarbonate Therapy**: Avoid bicarbonate for pH >6.9 unless there is severe acidosis or life-threatening conditions like arrhythmias.
- **Pitfall**: Do not administer insulin unless there is adequate fluid resuscitation and potassium levels are corrected if necessary.
- **HHS Management**:
    - **Fluids**: Initiate aggressive IV fluids with 0.9% NaCl and transition to a dextrose-containing solution once blood glucose levels approach 250 mg/dL to prevent hypoglycemia.
    - **Insulin**: Use a lower insulin infusion rate compared to DKA (0.05 units/kg/hr), as the primary issue in HHS is hyperosmolarity rather than ketosis.
    - **Pitfall**: Reassess and monitor frequently for potential complications like cerebral edema (more common in DKA but can occur in HHS with rapid fluid shifts).
- **Monitoring**: Regularly check blood glucose, electrolytes, anion gap, and arterial pH to assess treatment progress.

Relevant Guidelines

- The American Diabetes Association (ADA) guidelines

provide detailed protocols for the management of DKA and HHS, including fluid resuscitation, insulin therapy, and monitoring.

2. Adrenal Insufficiency And Thyroid Storm Management

Clinical Scenario
A 60-year-old male with a history of chronic adrenal insufficiency presents with confusion, hypotension, and fever. His serum cortisol is low (2 µg/dL), and his sodium is low (129 mEq/L), suggestive of an adrenal crisis.

Key Insight
Adrenal insufficiency and thyroid storm are life-threatening conditions that require urgent recognition and treatment.

Both conditions present with similar symptoms of shock, altered mental status, and dysregulated temperature, but treatment strategies differ significantly.

Tips and Pitfalls
- **Adrenal Insufficiency (Adrenal Crisis):**
    - **Hydrocortisone**: Administer IV hydrocortisone (100 mg) immediately, followed by 200 mg/day in divided doses. If there is no improvement, increase the dose.
    - **Fluids**: Start with aggressive IV fluids (normal saline or Ringer's lactate) to treat hypotension and dehydration.
    - **Pitfall**: Do not delay glucocorticoid replacement in the absence of lab confirmation—empiric treatment is crucial to avoid fatal consequences.

- **Monitor**: Frequently monitor electrolytes, especially sodium (which may be low due to aldosterone deficiency), and glucose.
- **Thyroid Storm**:
    - **Beta-blockers**: Administer propranolol (initial dose of 1–2 mg IV, then 1–3 mg every 6 hours) to control symptoms such as tachycardia and hypertension.
    - **Thionamides**: Start with propylthiouracil (PTU) or methimazole to inhibit thyroid hormone synthesis. PTU also inhibits the peripheral conversion of T4 to T3.
    - **Steroids**: Administer IV glucocorticoids (hydrocortisone 100 mg every 8 hours) to block the conversion of T4 to T3 and treat associated adrenal insufficiency.
    - **Pitfall**: Do not use iodine or radioactive iodine in the acute setting, as it can worsen the condition by increasing the release of thyroid hormones.
- **Monitoring**: Closely monitor for arrhythmias, as thyroid storm can lead to severe tachyarrhythmias, as well as renal function due to dehydration and shock.

Relevant Guidelines

- The American Association of Clinical Endocrinologists (AACE) provides recommendations for the diagnosis and management of adrenal insufficiency and thyroid storm, including the use of glucocorticoids and thionamides.

3. Pearls On Managing Blood Glucose In Critically Ill Patients

Clinical Scenario

A 70-year-old male with a history of hypertension, diabetes, and recent myocardial infarction is admitted to the ICU for respiratory failure. His blood glucose is consistently over 200 mg/dL, despite intermittent insulin administration.

Key Insight

Maintaining optimal blood glucose levels in critically ill patients is crucial for improving outcomes.

Hyperglycemia is associated with increased morbidity, while hypoglycemia can be equally dangerous, leading to neurologic injury and worsened prognosis.

Tight glucose control is necessary but must be balanced carefully.

Tips and Pitfalls

- **Target Blood Glucose**: The American Diabetes Association recommends a target blood glucose range of 140–180 mg/dL in critically ill patients, as evidence suggests that more aggressive control (<140 mg/dL) does not improve outcomes and increases the risk of hypoglycemia.
- **Insulin Protocols**: Use intravenous insulin infusion for precise control. Adjust the infusion rate based on frequent (every 1–2 hours) glucose monitoring.
  - **Pitfall**: Avoid abrupt cessation of insulin infusion—this can lead to rapid hyperglycemia. Use a transition strategy to subcutaneous insulin if the patient stabilizes.
- **Glucose Monitoring**: Check blood glucose levels frequently, ideally every 1–2 hours in the first 24–48 hours, and adjust insulin dosing accordingly.
- **Avoid Hypoglycemia**: Hypoglycemia (blood glucose <70 mg/dL) should be avoided at all costs, as it

increases the risk of adverse events. If hypoglycemia occurs, treat immediately with a rapid source of glucose (e.g., D50 solution) and reassess the insulin infusion rate.

- **Pitfall**: Over-correcting hyperglycemia by administering excess insulin can result in dangerous hypoglycemia, particularly in patients with renal failure or hepatic dysfunction.

Relevant Guidelines

- The NICE-SUGAR trial and the American College of Physicians (ACP) guidelines provide evidence-based strategies for blood glucose management in the ICU, emphasizing a moderate control approach with a range of 140–180 mg/dL.

CHAPTER 8: TRAUMA AND SURGICAL ICU MANAGEMENT

1. Pearls On Trauma Resuscitation And Damage Control Surgery

Clinical Scenario
A 32-year-old male is brought to the trauma bay after a high-speed motor vehicle collision. He is hypotensive (BP 80/50 mmHg), tachycardic (HR 125 bpm), and in respiratory distress. A primary survey reveals a suspected pelvic fracture, multiple rib fractures, and signs of internal bleeding. Initial resuscitation has failed to stabilize his vital signs.

Key Insight
Trauma resuscitation follows the ABCDE (Airway, Breathing, Circulation, Disability, Exposure) approach and focuses on immediate management of life-threatening injuries.

Damage control surgery (DCS) is a strategy aimed at stabilizing critically injured patients to prevent death from hemorrhagic shock and multi-organ failure, with definitive surgery planned once the patient is physiologically stable.

Tips and Pitfalls
- **Primary Survey**: Always begin with the ABCDE approach:
    - **Airway**: Secure the airway early, especially in patients with facial or neck injuries. Consider early intubation if there is any concern for

airway compromise.
- **Breathing**: Assess for pneumothorax or hemothorax and initiate rapid chest decompression or drainage as needed.
- **Circulation**: Use large-bore IV access or intraosseous access and initiate rapid fluid resuscitation. Use isotonic fluids (e.g., normal saline or lactated Ringer's) in the initial phase, followed by blood products (1:1:1 ratio of red blood cells, plasma, and platelets) as hemorrhagic shock persists.
- **Disability**: Assess neurological status using the Glasgow Coma Scale (GCS) and address any head injuries.
- **Exposure**: Remove all clothing to assess for hidden injuries, but avoid hypothermia.

- **Damage Control Surgery (DCS)**:
    - **Initial Surgery**: The goal of DCS is not to achieve definitive surgery but to control hemorrhage and stabilize the patient. This may include packing liver or splenic injuries, applying temporary vascular clamps, or controlling pelvic fractures with external fixation.
    - **Rewarm and Resuscitate**: Rewarm the patient during transport and resuscitation, as hypothermia impairs coagulation and worsens shock.
    - **Pitfall**: Avoid performing definitive repairs of major organ injuries (e.g., liver, spleen) in the first phase of resuscitation, as prolonged surgery can exacerbate coagulopathy and shock.

- **Post-Resuscitation**: After stabilization, definitive

surgery should be performed when the patient is hemodynamically stable and coagulopathy is corrected.

Relevant Guidelines
- The Advanced Trauma Life Support (ATLS) guidelines provide a standardized approach for trauma resuscitation and trauma surgery management, including the principles of damage control surgery and fluid resuscitation.

2. Managing Post-Operative Complications In The Icu

Clinical Scenario
A 60-year-old male with a history of hypertension and coronary artery disease undergoes a coronary artery bypass graft (CABG) surgery. Post-operatively, his condition deteriorates with increasing oxygen requirement, elevated lactate levels, and oliguria. He is transferred to the ICU for further management.

Key Insight
Post-operative complications can range from respiratory failure and infection to cardiovascular and renal dysfunction.
Early recognition and management are critical in preventing long-term morbidity or mortality. Multidisciplinary management, including frequent monitoring and timely interventions, is essential in the ICU.

Tips and Pitfalls
- **Respiratory Complications**:
    - **Ventilator Management**: Assess for postoperative atelectasis or pleural effusion,

which can worsen oxygenation. Early mobilization and the use of incentive spirometry can prevent complications.
- **Pitfall**: Avoid over-sedating patients, as this can delay weaning from the ventilator. Tailor sedation protocols to the patient's level of discomfort and physiological needs.

- **Cardiovascular Complications**:
  - **Monitoring Hemodynamics**: Post-cardiac surgery patients often experience hypotension or arrhythmias. Consider using a central venous catheter to monitor central venous pressure (CVP) and a pulmonary artery catheter for more accurate measurements in complex cases.
  - **Pitfall**: Hypotension in the post-operative phase may be due to factors other than blood loss (e.g., myocardial dysfunction, arrhythmias). Always assess for these causes.

- **Renal Complications**:
  - **Acute Kidney Injury (AKI)**: Monitor for AKI, especially in patients who have received nephrotoxic medications or have pre-existing renal conditions. Consider using diuretics cautiously and initiating renal replacement therapy if indicated.
  - **Pitfall**: Avoid unnecessary use of diuretics to treat oliguria, as this may worsen renal function.

- **Infection**:
  - **Surveillance for Infection**: Regularly monitor for signs of infection, including fever, elevated white blood cell count, or purulent discharge from surgical sites. Early

identification of infections allows for prompt antibiotic therapy.
- **Pitfall**: Avoid broad-spectrum antibiotics without culture data. Always narrow the spectrum based on susceptibility results.

Relevant Guidelines
- The Society of Critical Care Medicine (SCCM) provides guidelines for post-operative management in the ICU, with specific recommendations for monitoring hemodynamics, ventilation, and renal function.

3. Pearls On Anticoagulation Reversal In Bleeding Patients

Clinical Scenario
A 72-year-old male with atrial fibrillation and chronic anticoagulation therapy (warfarin) presents to the ICU with a large gastrointestinal bleed. His INR is elevated at 4.5, and his hemoglobin is dropping. He is hemodynamically unstable and requires urgent management to reverse his anticoagulation.

Key Insight
Reversing anticoagulation is crucial in the management of bleeding patients receiving oral anticoagulants or parenteral agents.

The approach varies based on the type of anticoagulant used, with specific reversal agents and strategies tailored to the individual anticoagulant.

Tips and Pitfalls
- **Warfarin Reversal**:
  - **Vitamin K**: Administer IV vitamin K (5–

10 mg) slowly over 30 minutes to reverse warfarin effects.
- **Prothrombin Complex Concentrates (PCC)**: If there is active bleeding or high-risk bleeding, consider using 4-factor PCC or fresh frozen plasma (FFP) to rapidly correct the INR.
- **Pitfall**: Avoid administering FFP alone for warfarin reversal, as it takes longer to correct the INR compared to PCC.

- **Direct Oral Anticoagulants (DOACs)**:
  - **Dabigatran (Direct Thrombin Inhibitor)**: Administer idarucizumab (Praxbind) for urgent reversal.
  - **Rivaroxaban and Apixaban (Factor Xa Inhibitors)**: For major bleeding, use Andexanet alfa or PCC.
  - **Pitfall**: DOAC reversal agents are expensive and not always available in all settings. In the absence of reversal agents, supportive care and hemodynamic stabilization are key, and strategies like dialysis may be used for dabigatran.

- **Unfractionated Heparin**:
  - **Protamine Sulfate**: Administer protamine sulfate for heparin reversal, using 1 mg of protamine per 100 units of heparin in the last dose.
  - **Pitfall**: Monitor for protamine-induced anaphylaxis or hypotension, especially in patients who have received high doses of heparin.

Relevant Guidelines

- The American College of Chest Physicians (CHEST) guidelines provide recommendations for anticoagulation management, including reversal strategies for warfarin, DOACs, and heparin in patients with major bleeding or requiring urgent surgery.

CHAPTER 9: NUTRITION AND METABOLISM

1. Early Enteral Nutrition: Benefits And Timing

Clinical Scenario
A 55-year-old woman is admitted to the ICU following a major abdominal surgery for a perforated diverticulum. She is stable post-operatively but has a nasogastric tube in place and is being considered for nutritional support. The team is debating whether to initiate enteral feeding immediately or wait a few days.

Key Insight
Early enteral nutrition (EN) is the preferred method of feeding for critically ill patients who are expected to have prolonged nutrition needs.

Initiating EN within 24–48 hours after admission to the ICU is associated with improved clinical outcomes, including decreased infection rates, fewer complications, and reduced length of ICU stay.

EN preserves gut integrity, reduces the risk of bacterial translocation, and supports immune function.

Tips and Pitfalls
- **Benefits of Early EN**:
    - **Gut Function**: Early enteral feeding helps maintain gut integrity by stimulating the mucosa and promoting motility. It also helps prevent the development of ileus and reduces

the risk of gut atrophy.
- **Reduced Infection Risk**: Enteral nutrition is associated with fewer infections (e.g., ventilator-associated pneumonia, catheter-related bloodstream infections) compared to parenteral nutrition.
- **Pitfall**: Avoid delaying EN in stable patients for fear of aspiration. Proper tube placement, patient positioning, and monitoring are essential.

- **Monitoring EN**:
  - **Tolerance**: Begin with a slow infusion and gradually increase the rate. Monitor for signs of intolerance, such as gastric residuals >500 ml, abdominal distension, or vomiting.
  - **Pitfall**: Aggressive feeding in the early days may lead to gastrointestinal complications (e.g., diarrhea, bloating), especially in critically ill patients with delayed gastric emptying or intestinal dysfunction.

- **Choosing Enteral Formulas**: Select appropriate formulas based on the patient's metabolic needs (e.g., high-protein formulas for patients with burns or trauma, specialized formulas for hepatic or renal failure).

Relevant Guidelines

- The European Society for Clinical Nutrition and Metabolism (ESPEN) and American Society for Parenteral and Enteral Nutrition (ASPEN) guidelines recommend initiating enteral feeding within 24–48 hours for most ICU patients, provided there are no contraindications (e.g., bowel obstruction, significant ileus).

2. Parenteral Nutrition: Indications And Complications

Clinical Scenario
A 60-year-old male with severe pancreatitis is admitted to the ICU. He has been NPO (nil per os) for several days, and his nutrition needs are not being met with enteral feeding due to gastric ileus. The team is considering initiating parenteral nutrition (PN) to provide essential nutrients.

Key Insight
Parenteral nutrition (PN) is indicated when enteral nutrition is contraindicated or not feasible.

While it provides critical nutrients, PN is associated with risks such as infections, liver dysfunction, and metabolic complications.

PN should only be initiated when necessary, and its duration should be as short as possible.

Tips and Pitfalls
- **Indications for PN**:
    - **Failure of Enteral Feeding**: In patients who cannot tolerate enteral nutrition (e.g., due to ileus, severe malabsorption, or gastrointestinal obstruction), PN may be required to meet nutritional needs.
    - **Critically Ill Patients**: If a patient is expected to be NPO for more than 7 days and enteral feeding is not possible, PN should be considered.
    - **Pitfall**: Avoid early initiation of PN unless enteral nutrition is absolutely

contraindicated. Early use of PN is associated with an increased risk of infections and complications.

- **PN Complications**:
  - **Infections**: Central venous catheter (CVC) infections are the most common complication of PN. Ensure proper technique during catheter insertion and maintenance, and avoid prolonged use of the same catheter.
  - **Metabolic Complications**: Hyperglycemia is a common issue, particularly in critically ill patients. Regular monitoring of blood glucose and insulin administration is required. Lipid overload can also result in hypertriglyceridemia.
  - **Liver Dysfunction**: Long-term PN can lead to liver dysfunction, including cholestasis and fatty liver disease. Regular liver function tests should be monitored during prolonged PN.
  - **Pitfall**: Never use peripheral veins for PN unless it is a short-term solution, as this increases the risk of thrombophlebitis and extravasation.

Relevant Guidelines

- The ASPEN and Society of Critical Care Medicine (SCCM) guidelines recommend PN only for patients who cannot receive enteral nutrition or when it is contraindicated. Monitoring for complications such as infection, metabolic derangements, and liver dysfunction is essential in patients on PN.

3. Metabolic Support In Critically Ill Patients

Clinical Scenario
A 70-year-old male is admitted to the ICU with severe sepsis and acute respiratory failure. His nutritional status is poor, and he is unable to tolerate enteral feeding. The team must decide on the appropriate metabolic support to provide during his recovery.

Key Insight
Metabolic support in critically ill patients includes both nutritional and non-nutritional strategies to address catabolism, provide energy, and support recovery.

Tailored approaches to metabolic support, including balancing energy intake and managing hyperglycemia, are essential in critically ill patients.

Tips and Pitfalls
- **Energy Requirements**:
    - **Nutritional Targets**: Critically ill patients have increased energy requirements due to the metabolic stress of illness. The goal is to provide enough calories to avoid catabolism while not overfeeding. Indirect calorimetry is the gold standard for measuring energy expenditure but is often not available. In its absence, predictive equations (e.g., the Harris-Benedict equation) can be used.
    - **Pitfall**: Avoid overfeeding patients, as excessive caloric intake can lead to complications such as hyperglycemia, fatty liver, and increased respiratory workload.
- **Protein Requirements**:
    - **Protein Needs**: Critically ill patients require higher protein intake to maintain muscle mass, support immune function, and

facilitate wound healing. Aim for 1.2–2.0 g/kg of body weight per day, depending on the severity of illness.
- **Pitfall**: Ensure protein delivery is adequate, but do not provide excessive protein, particularly in patients with renal dysfunction, as this can exacerbate kidney failure.
- **Electrolyte and Fluid Management**:
  - **Fluid Balance**: Critically ill patients often have significant fluid shifts and imbalances, including hypovolemia or fluid overload. Careful monitoring of fluid intake, output, and electrolytes (particularly sodium, potassium, calcium, and phosphate) is necessary.
  - **Pitfall**: Avoid rapid correction of electrolyte imbalances (especially sodium), as this can lead to complications such as central pontine myelinolysis.

Relevant Guidelines

- The ASPEN and SCCM guidelines emphasize the importance of providing individualized metabolic support based on energy expenditure, protein requirements, and fluid balance. They recommend early nutrition (enteral when possible) and personalized approaches to managing glucose and electrolytes in critically ill patients.

CHAPTER 10: ETHICAL AND END-OF-LIFE ISSUES

1. Discussing Goals Of Care With Families

Clinical Scenario
A 68-year-old man is admitted to the ICU after suffering a massive stroke, leaving him comatose with minimal neurological response. His family is uncertain about the next steps, and there is disagreement on whether aggressive treatment should continue or if comfort care should be considered.

Key Insight
Discussing goals of care with families is a cornerstone of managing critically ill patients, especially when prognosis is uncertain.

Clear, compassionate communication is essential in aligning treatment with the patient's values and wishes, ensuring that the family feels supported in making informed decisions.

It's important to initiate these discussions early to prevent decision fatigue and to clarify the patient's goals, especially in situations involving life-limiting illnesses.

Tips and Pitfalls
- **Start Early**:
    - Early conversations about goals of care can prevent escalation of interventions that may not align with the patient's wishes. It's important to assess the patient's baseline

functional status and values early in the ICU stay.
    - **Pitfall**: Avoid waiting until life-threatening complications occur before having these discussions, as this can create an emotional and time-sensitive pressure for families.
- **Use a Structured Approach**:
    - Utilize frameworks such as the **SPIKES protocol** (Setting, Perception, Invitation, Knowledge, Empathy, and Summary) to guide the conversation. This approach allows the physician to assess the family's understanding, express empathy, provide clear information, and involve them in decision-making.
    - **Pitfall**: Avoid medical jargon or overly technical explanations that can overwhelm the family. The goal is to make the discussion understandable and focused on the patient's preferences.
- **Respect Family Dynamics**:
    - Recognize that families may have different cultural, religious, and emotional responses to illness. Tailor the conversation to these differences and ensure that all relevant family members are included in the discussion.
    - **Pitfall**: Do not ignore family members who may be less vocal, as their perspectives and concerns are important in the decision-making process.

Relevant Guidelines

- The **American College of Physicians (ACP)** and

American Academy of Hospice and Palliative Medicine (AAHPM) recommend early, open discussions of prognosis and treatment goals in the ICU. These organizations emphasize the importance of providing families with honest, clear information about likely outcomes and treatment options to align care with the patient's values.

2. Pearls On Managing Withdrawal Of Life Support

Clinical Scenario
A 74-year-old woman with advanced metastatic cancer has been on mechanical ventilation for several days after respiratory failure. Despite aggressive treatment, her prognosis is poor, and her family has requested a discussion about the possibility of withdrawing life support.

Key Insight
Withdrawal of life support is a complex and emotionally charged process that requires careful management to ensure the patient's comfort, respect for their wishes, and support for the family.

The primary goal is to allow a natural death while alleviating suffering.

This process should be patient-centered, with the healthcare team providing clear guidance and offering compassionate support throughout.

Tips and Pitfalls
- **Confirm the Decision:**
    - Before proceeding, ensure that the decision to withdraw life support is in line with the patient's wishes (as documented in advance

directives or discussed with the family). If the patient has no advance directives, ensure that the family has a clear understanding of the prognosis and that the decision reflects their loved one's values.
- **Pitfall**: Avoid acting hastily in emotionally charged situations. Provide adequate time for the family to process the decision and ensure they are fully informed.

- **Sedation and Comfort**:
  - Administer appropriate sedation and analgesia to ensure that the patient is comfortable during the withdrawal process. Medications such as morphine or benzodiazepines are commonly used to alleviate distress and provide comfort.
  - **Pitfall**: Over-sedation or under-sedation can lead to either unnecessary suffering or an unintended hastening of death. Tailor the dose to the patient's needs and response.

- **Family Support**:
  - Ensure that the family is present during the withdrawal of life support, if they wish to be. Offer emotional support and ensure that they understand what to expect during the process.
  - **Pitfall**: Be mindful of the family's emotional responses, which may include grief, guilt, or uncertainty. Offer counseling or spiritual support as needed.

- **Timing and Process**:
  - Withdraw life support gradually when possible (e.g., reducing ventilator settings before extubation) to allow the patient to

transition peacefully. Monitor the patient closely to ensure they do not experience undue distress during the process.
- **Pitfall**: Don't rush the process or impose an artificial timeline. The goal is to allow the patient's body to die naturally while keeping them comfortable.

Relevant Guidelines
- The **American Thoracic Society** and **Society of Critical Care Medicine (SCCM)** provide guidelines on end-of-life care in the ICU, which include recommendations for ethical withdrawal of life support, focusing on compassionate communication, patient comfort, and supporting families through the process.

3. Navigating Ethical Dilemmas In The Icu

Clinical Scenario
A 42-year-old woman with severe alcoholic cirrhosis is admitted to the ICU with acute liver failure. She is comatose and requires mechanical ventilation. Her family insists on every possible intervention, but her prognosis is extremely poor, and the healthcare team is concerned about the futility of continued aggressive treatment.

Key Insight
ICU physicians often encounter ethical dilemmas when the balance between providing life-sustaining treatment and respecting the patient's dignity becomes unclear.

These situations require careful navigation, with an emphasis on communication, respect for patient autonomy, and ethical principles such as beneficence and non-maleficence.

When treatment options are limited or the prognosis is poor, healthcare teams should guide families toward decisions that align with the patient's values and avoid interventions that may cause unnecessary suffering.

Tips and Pitfalls
- **Futility of Treatment:**
  - In situations where further treatment is deemed futile, it's important to address this directly with the family, discussing the potential for harm or suffering. Be clear about the limitations of treatment and focus on quality of life rather than quantity of life.
  - **Pitfall:** Avoid the temptation to pursue aggressive interventions when they are unlikely to benefit the patient. Be honest and transparent about the prognosis and treatment options.
- **Ethical Principles in Practice:**
  - The principles of **autonomy** (respecting the patient's wishes), **beneficence** (acting in the patient's best interest), and **non-maleficence** (avoiding harm) should guide decision-making. Consider consulting ethics committees or palliative care specialists if the team is divided or if there is disagreement within the family.
  - **Pitfall:** Ethical dilemmas often arise when there is a disconnect between the patient's previously expressed wishes and the family's emotional responses. It's essential to mediate these situations with care and sensitivity.
- **Involving Multidisciplinary Teams:**
  - Involve social workers, chaplains, and

palliative care specialists to help navigate complex ethical discussions and provide additional support to both the patient and family.
    - **Pitfall**: Don't rely solely on the physician's perspective. A collaborative, team-based approach is essential when addressing ethical dilemmas in the ICU.

Relevant Guidelines

- The **SCCM's Ethics Committee** and **American Medical Association (AMA)** provide guidelines on ethical decision-making in critical care. These guidelines emphasize the importance of shared decision-making, the role of ethics committees, and the need for early and ongoing communication with patients and families.

CASE STUDIES IN ICU

Case 1: Acute Respiratory Distress Syndrome (Ards) In A Covid-19 Patient

Clinical Scenario
A 54-year-old male with COVID-19 is admitted to the ICU after developing severe ARDS. He is intubated, and despite mechanical ventilation, his oxygenation remains poor. The team is considering proning as a strategy to improve oxygenation.

Key Insight
Proning has been shown to improve oxygenation in patients with ARDS by improving ventilation-perfusion matching and reducing atelectasis.

However, it requires careful monitoring and proper technique to avoid complications.

Tips and Pitfalls
- **Tip**: Ensure that proning is done early in the course of ARDS when oxygenation is not improving with conventional mechanical ventilation. Keep the patient in the prone position for 12-16 hours at a time.
- **Pitfall**: Don't attempt proning without adequate staff and expertise; improper positioning can lead to pressure sores, airway displacement, and facial injury.

Relevant Guidelines

- The **Surviving Sepsis Campaign** guidelines recommend proning for patients with severe ARDS (PaO2/FiO2 < 150) who are receiving mechanical ventilation.

Case 2: Acute Pulmonary Embolism (Pe) In A Post-Surgical Patient

Clinical Scenario
A 72-year-old woman is recovering from hip replacement surgery and suddenly develops shortness of breath and chest pain. A CT pulmonary angiogram reveals a massive pulmonary embolism.

Key Insight
In the ICU, early identification and management of pulmonary embolism (PE) are critical.

Hemodynamic stability should guide treatment, with thrombolysis or surgical embolectomy considered for high-risk patients.

Tips and Pitfalls
- **Tip**: If the patient is hemodynamically unstable, administer thrombolytics (alteplase or tenecteplase) after ruling out contraindications. Anticoagulation with heparin is necessary for stable patients.
- **Pitfall**: Don't delay thrombolysis or embolectomy in a patient who is hemodynamically unstable. Waiting for imaging or lab results can be fatal.

Relevant Guidelines
- The **American College of Chest Physicians (ACCP)** guidelines recommend the use of thrombolytics in high-risk, hemodynamically unstable patients with

PE and the use of anticoagulation therapy in stable patients.

Case 3: Hypertensive Crisis In A Post-Cardiac Surgery Patient

Clinical Scenario
A 65-year-old male post-cardiac surgery develops a sudden increase in blood pressure (BP 210/130 mmHg), associated with agitation and acute kidney injury (AKI). He is in the ICU on a ventilator.

Key Insight
In post-operative cardiac surgery patients, hypertensive crises can lead to complications such as stroke, AKI, and myocardial ischemia.

The goal is to lower the blood pressure gradually to prevent further complications.

Tips and Pitfalls

- **Tip**: Use intravenous antihypertensives such as labetalol or nicardipine to gradually lower BP to avoid sudden drops. Target BP reduction should be 20-25% in the first hour.
- **Pitfall**: Avoid rapid BP reduction as it can precipitate organ ischemia, particularly in the brain and kidneys.

Relevant Guidelines

- The **American College of Cardiology (ACC)** and **American Heart Association (AHA)** guidelines recommend a gradual reduction of BP in hypertensive crises to avoid end-organ damage.

Case 4: Severe Hyperkalemia In A Patient With Acute Kidney Injury

Clinical Scenario
A 62-year-old diabetic patient with AKI develops severe hyperkalemia (K+ 7.2 mEq/L). The patient is lethargic and has an ECG showing peaked T-waves and a widened QRS complex.

Key Insight
Hyperkalemia is a life-threatening electrolyte abnormality.

Immediate interventions are required to stabilize the heart and shift potassium intracellularly, followed by measures to eliminate excess potassium.

Tips and Pitfalls
- **Tip**: Administer calcium gluconate to stabilize the cardiac membrane, followed by insulin and glucose to drive potassium into cells. Dialysis should be considered if renal function does not improve.
- **Pitfall**: Don't delay treatment based on laboratory results alone. Clinical signs such as ECG changes require immediate intervention.

Relevant Guidelines
- The **Kidney Disease: Improving Global Outcomes (KDIGO)** guidelines recommend emergent treatment with calcium, insulin, glucose, and/or dialysis for severe hyperkalemia.

Case 5: Diabetic Ketoacidosis (Dka) In An Icu Patient

Clinical Scenario
A 48-year-old woman with Type 1 diabetes is admitted to the ICU with DKA. She has been vomiting and has a blood glucose level of 450 mg/dL with a pH of 7.1.

Key Insight
Management of DKA in the ICU includes fluid resuscitation, insulin therapy, and electrolyte replacement.

Close monitoring of glucose and electrolytes is essential, especially potassium levels, as they can fluctuate rapidly during treatment.

Tips and Pitfalls
- **Tip**: Start insulin infusion after adequate fluid resuscitation and monitor potassium levels closely, correcting hypokalemia before starting insulin.
- **Pitfall**: Don't correct glucose too rapidly. Aim for a gradual decrease of 50-75 mg/dL per hour to prevent cerebral edema.

Relevant Guidelines
- The **American Diabetes Association (ADA)** guidelines recommend the use of an insulin infusion and careful management of fluids and electrolytes in DKA patients.

Case 6: Acute Pancreatitis In The Icu

Clinical Scenario
A 39-year-old woman with gallstone pancreatitis develops severe abdominal pain and hypotension. She is admitted to the ICU for supportive care.

Key Insight
Early supportive care is crucial in managing acute pancreatitis.

Fluid resuscitation is the cornerstone of treatment, and organ support may be required in severe cases. Monitoring for complications like infected pancreatic necrosis is essential.

Tips and Pitfalls
- **Tip**: Start aggressive intravenous fluid resuscitation with isotonic saline or Ringer's lactate. Use early enteral feeding if possible to reduce complications.
- **Pitfall**: Avoid the use of prophylactic antibiotics in the absence of infection, as this does not improve outcomes.

Relevant Guidelines
- The **American College of Gastroenterology (ACG)** guidelines recommend aggressive fluid resuscitation and early enteral nutrition for patients with acute pancreatitis.

Case 7: Septic Shock In An Immunocompromised Patient

Clinical Scenario
A 56-year-old male with leukemia develops septic shock after a

chemotherapy cycle. He presents with fever, hypotension, and a positive blood culture for E. coli.

Key Insight
Septic shock in immunocompromised patients requires early, broad-spectrum antibiotic therapy, aggressive fluid resuscitation, and hemodynamic support.

Prompt recognition and intervention are crucial to reduce mortality.

Tips and Pitfalls
- **Tip**: Administer broad-spectrum antibiotics immediately after blood cultures are drawn. Early vasopressor support may be required if the patient remains hypotensive after fluid resuscitation.
- **Pitfall**: Don't wait for culture results before starting antibiotics in septic shock. Delay in antibiotic administration increases mortality risk.

Relevant Guidelines
- The **Surviving Sepsis Campaign** guidelines emphasize early recognition and treatment of septic shock, including broad-spectrum antibiotics and timely hemodynamic support.

Case 8: Status Epilepticus In An Icu Patient

Clinical Scenario
A 70-year-old woman with a history of stroke presents to the ICU with continuous generalized seizures lasting for 10 minutes. She is intubated and on mechanical ventilation.

Key Insight

Status epilepticus is a neurological emergency that requires rapid intervention to prevent brain damage.

First-line treatments include benzodiazepines followed by antiepileptic drugs (AEDs) if seizures persist.

Tips and Pitfalls

- **Tip**: Administer lorazepam or diazepam intravenously for immediate seizure control. If seizures persist, follow with phenytoin or levetiracetam.
- **Pitfall**: Don't wait for laboratory results before treating. Status epilepticus is a medical emergency that requires immediate action.

Relevant Guidelines

- The **American Epilepsy Society (AES)** recommends benzodiazepines as the first-line treatment for status epilepticus, followed by second-line AEDs if seizures persist.

Case 9: Acute Myocardial Infarction (Mi) In The Icu

Clinical Scenario
A 68-year-old man with a history of coronary artery disease presents with chest pain, sweating, and ST-segment elevation on ECG. He is admitted to the ICU for monitoring and management after thrombolysis.

Key Insight
In the ICU, the management of acute myocardial infarction (MI) involves monitoring for complications like arrhythmias, heart failure, and recurrent ischemia.

Antiplatelet therapy, anticoagulation, and beta-blockers are key components of treatment.

Tips and Pitfalls

- **Tip**: Administer dual antiplatelet therapy and anticoagulants. Consider initiating beta-blockers if there are no contraindications (e.g., hypotension or bradycardia).
- **Pitfall**: Avoid aggressive fluid resuscitation in the early stages of MI, as this can worsen heart failure.

Relevant Guidelines

- The **AHA/ACC** guidelines recommend early reperfusion with thrombolytics or percutaneous coronary intervention and the use of antiplatelet agents in patients with ST-segment elevation MI.

Case 10: Brain Death Determination In An Icu Patient

Clinical Scenario
A 50-year-old man is admitted to the ICU following a traumatic brain injury. Despite maximal support, he has no brainstem reflexes, no spontaneous respiration, and no response to pain. The team is considering brain death determination.

Key Insight
Brain death determination requires two clinical examinations and confirmatory tests.

The process is emotionally difficult but must follow strict legal and medical criteria to ensure that the diagnosis is accurate and ethical.

Tips and Pitfalls
- **Tip**: Ensure that all confounding factors (e.g., hypothermia, drug intoxication) have been ruled out before brain death testing. Document all assessments meticulously.
- **Pitfall**: Don't rush the determination of brain death; this process requires time and thorough documentation. Inaccurate testing can lead to misdiagnosis.

Relevant Guidelines
- The **American Academy of Neurology (AAN)** guidelines provide criteria for determining brain death, including clinical examination, apnea testing, and confirmatory tests such as cerebral blood flow

studies.

ABOUT THE AUTHOR

Dr Essam Abdelhakim

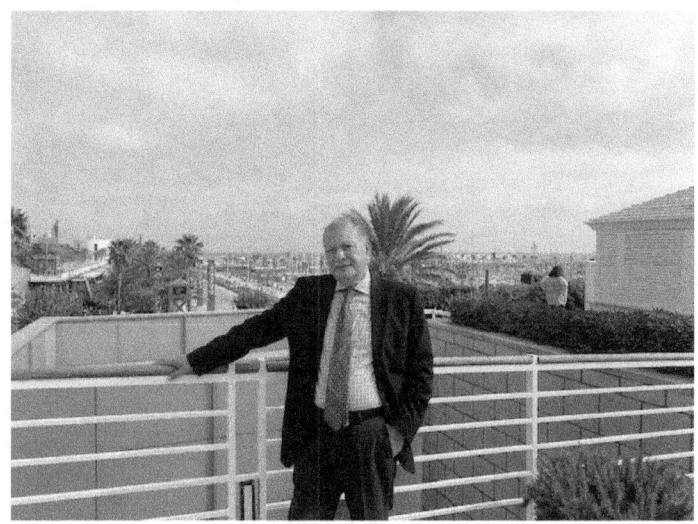

Senior Consultant and Expert in Medical Education

www.ingramcontent.com/pod-product-compliance
Lightning Source LLC
Chambersburg PA
CBHW071109240526
45469CB00006BD/2407